Essential Oils

30 Recipes For The Entire Family

Table of content

Introduction

There you are, standing in the cold and flu aisle once again, trying to decide what remedy you want to get for your ailing little one. You read the warnings, you try to read the ingredient list, and you wish there was a natural option you could use for your child.

Something that would help ease the aches and pains, and something that you didn't have to have a degree from Harvard to pronounce.

Thankfully, there is. For years upon years, essential oils have been used to help with symptoms from all kinds of illnesses and ailments, and you can use them today. Not just for the flu and cold, either.

You can ease the pain of tooth aches, stomach aches, and head aches, just to name a few. Aches not an issue for you? What about sleeping and stress? With essential oils, you have a natural way to help you fall asleep, stay asleep, and wake up feeling refreshed. You can drip a few drops into a diffuser or a warmer, and invite the lush smell to fill your home and bring you and your family so much relaxation, homework will be a breeze.

Essential oils are things that are tried and true. You know how high your standards are for your own health and comfort and for the health and comfort for your entire family, and essential oils live up to those standards.

They wouldn't be the one thing that has stood the test of time, above all other home remedies that have been known to man if they didn't bring the results that you want. They are made from all of the plants you see around you, nature's remedies.

This planet is full of everything you need to be healthy and happy, and most of that is growing right beneath our feet. So what are you waiting for? You know you would give anything to ensure the health and happiness of your home, and with nothing more than a few drops of oil, you can.

These oils are going to change your life, and you are going to fall in love with the results. No more standing in the cold and flu aisle. No more hoping that you can unwind enough to fall asleep tonight. No more stress.

These oils are just what you have been looking for, so go ahead, change your life for good.

Chapter 1 – Just the Essentials

If you have ever heard the phrase "get back to the basics of life", you know how essential those little things you tend to every day are. You may not think of them when you are doing them, you may not be thanked for the time and work you put into doing them, but at the end of the day, if they didn't get done, everyone would notice.

Just like you rise up and take care of the essentials, these oils have come along to take care of you. Toss a few drops in your diffuser, warm a few drops in your warmer, or mix with the carrier oil of your choice, and apply to your forehead or behind your ears.

Any way you choose to indulge in these oils, you are going to get the benefits you hope for. These oils are exactly what you need to brighten up your day and get ready to get things done.

The Good Day Blend

10 drops chamomile

12 drops bergamot

6 drops grapefruit

Mix oils together, and store in an oil jar. You can toss in your diffuser or mix a few drops to place in your oil warmer. Either way plug in your device and enjoy the wonderful scent that fills your home.

When you let this oil blend fill your home, not only are you creating a fresh, sweet scent that is going to put everyone in a good mood, but you are creating an atmosphere that brings out peace and tranquility in everyone that resides there.

Your house is already a safe haven for your friends and family, why not make it a calming oasis, too?

Get ready to present a slice of heaven on earth with this incredible blend of oils. Have a good day!

Happiness

12 drops sunflower oil

12 drops cedar

12 drops rose

12 drops lilac oil

Mix oils together, and store in an oil jar. You can toss in your diffuser or mix a few drops to place in your oil warmer. Either way plug in your device and enjoy the wonderful scent that fills your home.

Few things are able to bring happiness into your day like a summer day can. Through the long winters we all look forward to those bright, sunny days, and with these oils burning in the background of your home, you can have just that.

Get ready for a freshness that brings out the best in everyone that breathes it in, and have happiness abound everywhere in your home.

Meadows and Flowers

10 drops rose oil

10 drops lemongrass

5 drops cedar

Mix oils together, and store in an oil jar. You can toss in your diffuser or mix a few drops to place in your oil warmer. Either way plug in your device and enjoy the wonderful scent that fills your home.

Think of taking a stroll through a field of wild flowers on the edge of a mystic wood, and you are in for the calming effect of your life. Use this blend daily for the best relaxation you can imagine.

The Focus

5 drops ginger

5 drops basil oil

10 drops grapefruit oil

Mix oils together, and store in an oil jar. You can toss in your diffuser or mix a few drops to place in your oil warmer. Either way plug in your device and enjoy the wonderful scent that fills your home.

This is a light and fresh blend that will bring your mind to attention faster than a general in the army could. Use in your diffuser for an all over scent, or blend with a carrier oil and spread on your forehead for a more concentrated result.

Concentrated application for concentration... what could be better than that?

Perfection in a Bottle

5 drops tea tree oil

5 drops peppermint oil

5 drops ginger oil

5 drops cedar oil

5 drops cypress oil

Mix oils together, and store in an oil jar. You can toss in your diffuser or mix a few drops to place in your oil warmer. Either way plug in your device and enjoy the wonderful scent that fills your home.

Clarity, energy, focus... a great combination for anyone in any stage of life. This is the blend you need to start your day, no matter what your day holds in store for you.

Please note:

There are mixed opinions on whether or not you should ingest essential oils. Some people say it's just fine, others swear that it's toxic and you should avoid it at all costs.

You can make your own decisions, but remember that if you do decide to ingest them, you need to highly dilute the oil you are ingesting, and only take 1 or 2 drops in an entire day. Never consume more than this, and never let children under the age of 18 ingest oils at all.

They are full of wonderful benefits, but they need to be treated the right way, and moderation and respect are 2 of the biggest essentials that come with the use of essential oils.

Chapter 2 – For the Grown Ups

Mom and Dad certainly need to do their part when it comes to staying healthy, and that can be a bit of a challenge when you are busy running errands, working, and minding the children.

Energy, sleep, and relaxation seem to be distant memories in your busy life, but with the help of these essential oils, you are going to get a glimpse of that back. Use these oils in a diffuser, in an oil warmer, or mixed with a carrier oil for the best results, and get ready to feel like you again.

Have you missed those nights when you felt like you could go on forever? Do you miss those mornings when you get up and get right to work, ready to take on the day? If you do, then these are the oils for you.

It doesn't take long before you see the results of them in your life. Sleeping better, thinking more clearly, and focusing on what you need to do are just the beginning. Soon, you are going to see more energy and better health tag along, too!

The Energizer Deluxe

10 drops ginger oil

12 drops cinnamon oil

12 drops garlic oil

Mix oils together, and store in an oil jar. You can toss in your diffuser or mix a few drops to place in your oil warmer. Either way plug in your device and enjoy the wonderful scent that fills your home.

This rich blend of oils is the perfect spice you need to fire up your day and get going. If you need that extra burst, mix with a carrier oil of your choice and drop a few drops on your chest or jacket.

The fresh scent is going to keep you going, long after your morning coffee wears off.

The Friday Night Special

5 drops rose oil

5 drops chamomile

Mix oils together, and store in an oil jar. You can toss in your diffuser or mix a few drops to place in your oil warmer. Either way plug in your device and enjoy the wonderful scent that fills your home.

At the end of a long work week, sitting down and relaxing is the top priority for anyone. And this oil is going to help you wash away the stress of the work week you just completed, and set you up for a weekend of relaxation and rejuvenation.

Clear Mind and Soul

10 drops argon oil

12 drops frankincense oil

5 drops cypress oil

Mix oils together, and store in an oil jar. You can toss in your diffuser or mix a few drops to place in your oil warmer. Either way plug in your device and enjoy the wonderful scent that fills your home.

Warm this oil if you need to focus and pay attention to the task at hand. It is the perfect blend, making you feel relaxed, yet alert and ready to take on whatever challenge you need to face.

Good Night's Sleep

10 drops lavender oil

5 drops rose

Mix oils together, and store in an oil jar. You can toss in your diffuser or mix a few drops to place in your oil warmer. Either way plug in your device and enjoy the wonderful scent that fills your home.

Get this going in your diffuser about half an hour before you get ready for bed. By the time you are ready to go, your room is going to be filled with this relaxing scent, and you will crawl into your bed, and be transported to a wonderful, restful dreamland.

Tranquil Blast

10 drops chamomile

10 drops Bergamot

10 drops orange oil

10 drops cypress oil

10 drops frankincense

Mix oils together, and store in an oil jar. You can toss in your diffuser or mix a few drops to place in your oil warmer. Either way plug in your device and enjoy the wonderful scent that fills your home.

There is a lot of goodness squished into this tiny blend. When you burn this in your warmer, you are going to release into your home a blast of tranquility that will send you warm wishes and happiness all evening long.

Chapter 3 – For the Kids

We all want our kids to be happy, healthy, and well rested. Unfortunately, kids don't to go to bed on time, and they are always being exposed to all kinds of germs when they are at school or out with their friends.

If you have these blends handy, you are ready for anything. Burn in a warmer, let sit in a diffuser, or mix with a carrier oil and spread across your little one's forehead and you are protecting them from all kinds of germs.

The more natural you can get with your children, the happier you are going to be. You can give them all kinds of excellent benefits and never have to purchase anything that isn't natural. These oil blends were designed with your little ones in mind, and you are going to be pleased with the results.

They also have a sweet smell that will calm your little angel and help them get that good night's sleep you want them to get, making them ready for anything that comes their way!

Fairy Blend

10 drops rose oil

10 drops orange oil

5 drops tangerine oil

Mix oils together, and store in an oil jar. You can toss in your diffuser or mix a few drops to place in your oil warmer. Either way plug in your device and enjoy the wonderful scent that fills your home.

This is the perfect blend to use in the morning as you are getting your little one ready for the day. Wake them up the right way with this scent filling the home, bringing your little one right out of dream land and launching them into the mindset to face the day.

School is going to be a breeze when they wake up to this oil in your home.

Lemon Drops and Gum Drops

10 drops lemon oil

10 drops blue yarrow oil

Mix oils together, and store in an oil jar. You can toss in your diffuser or mix a few drops to place in your oil warmer. Either way plug in your device and enjoy the wonderful scent that fills your home.

This light and fresh scent is going to relax both of you after a long day of school.

Minty Magic

10 drops lemon

15 drops peppermint

5 drops tangerine

Mix oils together, and store in an oil jar. You can toss in your diffuser or mix a few drops to place in your oil warmer. Either way plug in your device and enjoy the wonderful scent that fills your home.

Mint clears the mind and tangerine soothes the soul. With this blend, you can both have a great day full of smiles and laughter.

Hugs and Kisses

10 drops roman chamomile

10 drops tangerine

5 drops orange

Mix oils together, and store in an oil jar. You can toss in your diffuser or mix a few drops to place in your oil warmer. Either way plug in your device and enjoy the wonderful scent that fills your home.

Mother's Perfect Blend

5 drops lavender

5 drops cypress

5 drops blue tansy

5 drops marjoram

Mix oils together, and store in an oil jar. You can toss in your diffuser or mix a few drops to place in your oil warmer. Either way plug in your device and enjoy the wonderful scent that fills your home.

This is truly the perfect blend no matter what you need for your child. Whether they have a bee sting, a skinned knee, a headache, or anything else, just mix with a carrier oil and apply gently.

Using this blend is a warmer is going to fill your home with a sweet smell that brings out a lot of happiness and giggles.

Please note:

There are a lot of mixed opinions when it comes to ingesting essential oils, but for children, all of the opinions are the same. Children should never ingest any essential oils for any reason. They can cause a lot of illness and toxicity in a child well into their teen years.

Always keep your oils diluted and out of reach, just for extra precaution when you have children around, and never let them ingest any of the oils, not even a single drop.

Chapter 4 – Illnesses and Pains

Illness likes to sneak up on the best of us, and in spite of all the precautions you take, you will have to deal with colds and flus from time to time. When that happens, have these remedies on hand, and you are ready for anything!

You can go to the store with confidence, not have to worry about your kids at school, and be able to get through your day with the knowledge that you have your immune system up and germs held at bay with the use of your essential oils.

Not only can you use with a diffuser, you can also add any of these oils to your soap for that added germ fighting benefit. This is your key to killing those germs and cutting back on those sick days! Say goodbye to the aches and pains and hello to sleep and comfort when you use these oil blends.

Place a few drops in your diffuser, oil warmer, or mix with a carrier oil to place on the forehead or tummy. Don't ingest these oils, but rather put them just on the head or stomach with carrier oils.

Coconut oil and baby oil are the best to use when you are dealing with illness. The added freshness to either one of them is going to help clear your mind and get you back up on your feet in no time.

The Cold Buster

10 drops lemon oil

10 drops eucalyptus oil

5 drops sage oil

Mix oils together, and store in an oil jar. You can toss in your diffuser or mix a few drops to place in your oil warmer. Either way plug in your device and enjoy the wonderful scent that fills your home.

You can also mix with a carrier oil, such as baby oil, and spread across your child's forehead or behind their ears to add potency to the blend.

The Flu Fighter

10 drops lemon oil

10 drops thyme oil

10 drops eucalyptus oil

10 drops spearmint oil

Mix oils together, and store in an oil jar. You can toss in your diffuser or mix a few drops to place in your oil warmer. Either way plug in your device and enjoy the wonderful scent that fills your home.

You know your child feels miserable, and you want nothing more than to scare that flu bug right out of them. With this blend, you are going to do just that, and in a matter of hours, too.

Mix with a carrier oil and apply to their forehead if you need to have that extra potency.

The Tummy Ache Fixer Upper

10 drops peppermint oil

10 drops spearmint oil

Mix oils together, and store in an oil jar. You can toss in your diffuser or mix a few drops to place in your oil warmer. Either way plug in your device and enjoy the wonderful scent that fills your home.

The minty freshness of this blend is going to clear out sinuses, and for the toughest of tummy aches, mix with a carrier oil and spread a few drops on your stomach. This is also gentle enough to use on your child's tummy if they are feeling ill as well.

The Magical Mix

10 drops bergamot oil

10 drops saffron oil

5 drops peppermint oil

Mix oils together, and store in an oil jar. You can toss in your diffuser or mix a few drops to place in your oil warmer. Either way plug in your device and enjoy the wonderful scent that fills your home.

The spicy scent of this oil mixed with the minty character is going to help you and your child relax, making it easier to fall asleep and fight off the illness that is holding on.

If you need a more potent exposure, mix a few drops with baby oil and apply to your forehead and chest.

The Clear Mind and Head Mix

5 drops tea tree oil

5 drops spearmint oil

5 drops peppermint oil

5 drops chamomile oil

Mix oils together, and store in an oil jar. You can toss in your diffuser or mix a few drops to place in your oil warmer. Either way plug in your device and enjoy the wonderful scent that fills your home.

You can also mix with a carrier oil and spread a few drops across your forehead to help you relax faster and gain a deeper experience with the oils. Coconut oil is a great carrier oil for this blend.

Chapter 5 – Sweet Dreams

These are the best blends to use for stress reduction as well as sleep. I highly recommend you mix up any of these batches and put them in your diffuser or oil warmer before you go to bed.

We all want to get that elusive good night's sleep, and with the world we live in, getting enough sleep, quality sleep, or sleep at all is a challenge. These oils are going to help you get what you want out of your rest, and feel ready to face the day again. Don't dread the morning, face it head on with a restful night's sleep at your back.

If you are using an oil warmer, make sure it is one that plugs in as you don't want a fire hazard. Place just a few drops in your diffuser and let the sweet smelling aromas fill the air. In no time at all you are going to feel relaxed, stress free, and able to fall asleep.

These oils work double duty. They not only help you fall asleep in the first place, but they are there to help you stay asleep and wake up feeling well rested and ready to face your day.

The Night Owl

15 drops

5 drops lemongrass

Mix oils together, and store in an oil jar. You can toss in your diffuser or mix a few drops to place in your oil warmer. Either way plug in your device and enjoy the wonderful scent that fills your home.

Goodnight Meadow

10 drops rosewood oil

5 drops lavender oil

5 drops rose oil

Mix oils together, and store in an oil jar. You can toss in your diffuser or mix a few drops to place in your oil warmer. Either way plug in your device and enjoy the wonderful scent that fills your home.

If you are having a night that is very difficult to sleep, mix this oil with a carrier oil (we recommend you use bedtime baby oil) and place a drop on your forehead and behind each of your ears.

The calming effect is incredible, and you will fall asleep quickly and reach a deeper, more relaxing sleep through the night.

The Dream Catcher

5 drops chamomile oil

5 drops

5 drops

Mix oils together, and store in an oil jar. You can toss in your diffuser or mix a few drops to place in your oil warmer. Either way plug in your device and enjoy the wonderful scent that fills your home.

Restful Drops

10 drops cardamom

8 drops frankincense

8 drops lavender oil

Mix oils together, and store in an oil jar. You can toss in your diffuser or mix a few drops to place in your oil warmer. Either way plug in your device and enjoy the wonderful scent that fills your home.

Deep Sleep

10 drops lavender

10 drops myrrh

Mix oils together, and store in an oil jar. You can toss in your diffuser or mix a few drops to place in your oil warmer. Either way plug in your device and enjoy the wonderful scent that fills your home.

This warm and woodsy scent is sure to take you to the deepest sleep you can imagine, say hello to those sweet dreams!

Chapter 6 – All the Rest

You take care of yourself, your partner, and the children, but what about the rest of the house? There's cleaning, laundry, air freshening, and all kinds of things that need to be done, and you are the one that has to do them!

With these oils, cleaning is going to be a synch. All you have to do is mix some of these blends, dilute with water, and get to your cleaning! It's that easy to use natural remedies to clean any mess.

Whether you are looking at a pile of laundry that needs to be washed, a bathroom that needs to be freshened, or a floor that you need to mop, essential oils are there to help.

Say goodbye to the dirt, smells, and germs when you use any one of these blends. Embrace the power of an essential clean, and never go back to the store bought chemical cleaners again.

The Drama Clean

10 drops tea tree oil

10 drops orange oil

10 drops spearmint oil

Mix oils together, and store in an oil jar. You can toss in your diffuser or mix a few drops to place in your oil warmer. Either way plug in your device and enjoy the wonderful scent that fills your home.

The citrus provides a nice burst of freshness, and there is cleaning properties to tea tree oil, so go ahead and use this on any area in your home that you want to clean and sanitize... a win all around!

Laundry Goddess

10 drops lavender

10 drops lemon

10 drops orange

Mix oils together, and store in an oil jar. When you do laundry, mix a few drops in with the laundry detergent of your choice, and watch the magi happen!

The Wonder Mix

5 drops tea tree oil

5 drops rose oil

10 drops sunflower oil

Mix oils together, and store in an oil jar. You can toss in your diffuser or mix a few drops to place in your oil warmer. Either way plug in your device and enjoy the wonderful scent that fills your home.

Citrus Burst

5 drops lemon oil

5 drops orange oil

5 drops blood orange oil

5 drops tea tree oil

Mix oils together, and store in an oil jar. You can toss in your diffuser or mix a few drops to place in your oil warmer. Either way plug in your device and enjoy the wonderful scent that fills your home.

As a cleaning agent, mix with water and put in a spray bottle. Spray on the area you want clean and mop up with a duster.

The Fresh Air Blend

10 drops lemon oil

15 drops lemongrass oil

5 drops peppermint

Mix oils together, and store in an oil jar. You can toss in your diffuser or mix a few drops to place in your oil warmer. Either way plug in your device and enjoy the wonderful scent that fills your home.

Conclusion

There you have it, everything you need to know about essential oils, and how to bring them into your life. As you can see, this is an easy and stress free way to incorporate a natural stress reducer, making it even easier for you to keep your family in the best of health.

If you struggle with body aches, pains, falling asleep, sleeping well, stress, or weight loss... you have found exactly what you need to make all of those things change for the better. Remember that you need to stick with this, and keep it going if you want to see all of the benefits.

Just like the standard medication we use today, you are going to feel some of the effects right away, but there are others that you have to see over time. But, the good news is that this is going to bring about all of those changes, and more! The wonderful thing about essential oils is that you get all of the benefits, even if you are only looking for one.

The same oil is going to relax you and get rid of stress as the oil that is going to help you fall asleep. The same oil that is good for your skin and hair is going to also keep your immune system up. You can't get away from the wonderful things these oils do for you, and as soon as you see the results for yourself, you won't even want to get away from them

So have fun and explore all of your essential oil options, and see what you can do for yourself and your family today!